# UNLOCKING WEIGHT LOSS

A Comprehensive Guide To Weight Loss Medication

By **Kelly Adams, RN**
Integrative Nutrition Health Coach

## Dedicated

To my incredible parents, Clement Gresham Jr. and Thelma Dade,

Your unwavering love, encouragement, and belief in me have shaped every step of my journey. Your resilience, hard work, and boundless support have been my greatest inspiration. You have always seen my potential, even when I doubted myself, and your faith in me has given me the strength to accomplish what once felt impossible.

This book is a reflection of the values you instilled in me - the desire to help others, the commitment to perseverance, and the belief that anything is possible with dedication and heart.

I am forever grateful to you both. This is for you!

With all my **love**,

*Kelly*

Copyright © 2025 by Kelly Adams
Published by Thriving Lifetime LLC
All rights reserved.

No portion of this publication can be reproduced in any form without written permission from the publisher or author, except as permitted by U.S. copyright law.

Information on weight loss medications is contained in this book. Obesity is a chronic disease. Medications can be part of a comprehensive treatment plan.

The history of weight loss medications is, with past use of dangerous substances. Today, a cautious approach is needed. Individuals considering these medications must meet specific criteria and undergo a medical assessment.

Various medications are explored, such as Orlistat, Phentermine, Qsymia, Contrave, Saxenda, Wegovy, and Zepbound, detailing their mechanisms, usage, side effects, weight loss potential, cost, and use in children. Common side effects include digestive issues, nervous system effects, and cardiovascular effects.

This book provides ways to manage side effects, emphasizing communication with healthcare providers and lifestyle modifications. Off-label medications like Bupropion and Metformin require careful consideration and monitoring. Compounding pharmacies offer some options but could carry risks.

Tips for discussing weight loss medications with healthcare providers are included to help encourage informed decision-making.

**Disclaimer:** This publication provides general information and is not a substitute for professional advice. While efforts have been made to ensure accuracy, the publisher and author make no warranties, expressed or implied. The information may not be suitable for your specific circumstances. Consult with a qualified professional for personalized advice. The publisher and author shall not be liable for any damages from using this information.

Book Cover by Raymond Adams

Photos by Kelly Adams & Raymond Adams

1st Edition 2025

ISBN: 979-8-9923318-3-7

# Table of Contents

**Introduction:** A Journey from Struggle to Cure..................

**UNLOCKING WEIGHT LOSS:**
A Comprehensive Guide to Weight Loss Medication..........1

## History Of Weight Loss Medications: ..........................3
- 1800s-1930s: Thyroid Extracts and Laxatives.......................3
- 1930s-1950s: Dinitrophenol and Amphetamines.................3
- 1950s-1970s: Appetite Suppressants........................................3
- 1980s-2000s: Fen-Phen and Its Aftermath.............................3
- 2000s-Present: New Generations and Mechanisms..............4
- Future Directions.............................................................................4

## Criteria for Considering Weight Loss Medications...5

## Medical Assessment Involve in Prescribing Weight Loss Medications....................7

## Making Informed Decisions Before Receiving Weight Loss Medications................8

## Understanding Obesity and Its Health Risks.............9

## Weight Loss Medications...........................................12

### Orlistat (Xenical, Alli)...........................................12
- History and FDA Approval...............................................12
- Mechanism of Action........................................................12
- Usage........................................................................................13
- Dosing......................................................................................13
- Side Effects.............................................................................13
- Weight Loss Potential........................................................13
- Cost...........................................................................................14
- Use in Children....................................................................14

### Phentermine (Adipex, Lomaira).......................15
- History and FDA Approval...............................................15
- Mechanism of Action........................................................15
- Usage........................................................................................16
- Dosing......................................................................................16
- Side Effects.............................................................................17
- Weight Loss Potential........................................................17
- Cost...........................................................................................18
- Use in Children....................................................................18

# Table of Contents

**Introduction:** A Journey from Struggle to Cure...................

## UNLOCKING WEIGHT LOSS:
A Comprehensive Guide to Weight Loss Medication..........1

### History Of Weight Loss Medications:........................3
- 1800s-1930s: Thyroid Extracts and Laxatives....................3
- 1930s-1950s: Dinitrophenol and Amphetamines.................3
- 1950s-1970s: Appetite Suppressants.....................................3
- 1980s-2000s: Fen-Phen and Its Aftermath............................3
- 2000s-Present: New Generations and Mechanisms..............4
- Future Directions....................................................................4

### Criteria for Considering Weight Loss Medications...5

### Medical Assessment Involve
in Prescribing Weight Loss Medications.....................7

### Making Informed Decisions
Before Receiving Weight Loss Medications...............8

### Understanding Obesity and Its Health Risks.............9

### Weight Loss Medications...........................................12

#### Orlistat (Xenical, Alli).........................................12
- History and FDA Approval..................................................12
- Mechanism of Action...........................................................12
- Usage......................................................................................13
- Dosing....................................................................................13
- Side Effects............................................................................13
- Weight Loss Potential...........................................................13
- Cost........................................................................................14
- Use in Children.....................................................................14

#### Phentermine (Adipex, Lomaira).......................15
- History and FDA Approval..................................................15
- Mechanism of Action...........................................................15
- Usage......................................................................................16
- Dosing....................................................................................16
- Side Effects............................................................................17
- Weight Loss Potential...........................................................17
- Cost........................................................................................18
- Use in Children.....................................................................18

# Table of Contents

**Introduction:** A Journey from Struggle to Cure..................

## UNLOCKING WEIGHT LOSS:
### A Comprehensive Guide to Weight Loss Medication..........1

### History Of Weight Loss Medications:........................3
- 1800s-1930s: Thyroid Extracts and Laxatives.....................3
- 1930s-1950s: Dinitrophenol and Amphetamines..................3
- 1950s-1970s: Appetite Suppressants.....................................3
- 1980s-2000s: Fen-Phen and Its Aftermath............................3
- 2000s-Present: New Generations and Mechanisms...............4
- Future Directions................................................................4

### Criteria for Considering Weight Loss Medications...5

### Medical Assessment Involve in Prescribing Weight Loss Medications....................7

### Making Informed Decisions Before Receiving Weight Loss Medications...............8

### Understanding Obesity and Its Health Risks.............9

### Weight Loss Medications...........................................12

#### Orlistat (Xenical, Alli).........................................12
- History and FDA Approval..................................................12
- Mechanism of Action...........................................................12
- Usage....................................................................................13
- Dosing...................................................................................13
- Side Effects...........................................................................13
- Weight Loss Potential..........................................................13
- Cost.......................................................................................14
- Use in Children....................................................................14

#### Phentermine (Adipex, Lomaira).......................15
- History and FDA Approval..................................................15
- Mechanism of Action...........................................................15
- Usage....................................................................................16
- Dosing...................................................................................16
- Side Effects...........................................................................17
- Weight Loss Potential..........................................................17
- Cost.......................................................................................18
- Use in Children....................................................................18

## Introduction:
## A Journey from Struggle to Cure

Welcome! My name is Kelly Adams, and this book is not just a narrative; it's an exploration, a guide, to weight loss medications.

For years, I struggled with my weight, a continual battle that many of you know all too well. The journey was filled with highs of brief successes and the lows of repeated setbacks. I tried everything: diets, surgery, exercise routines promising miraculous results, and holistic approaches to a more natural pathway. I also made use of personal trainers. In spite of my efforts, the scale barely budged, and my health continued to diminish.

The turning point came when I discovered weight-loss medications. Initially I was very skeptical. I researched, consulted medical professionals, and decided to try it. The results were miraculous. Not only did the numbers on the scale change, but my entire outlook on life transformed.

In this book, I will share everything I learned during my journey from the basic mechanisms of different medications, and how they work to the practical aspects of navigating this path with your healthcare provider. This book is not boring facts on weight loss medication. It's for those who have experienced unsuccessful attempts at losing weight, healthcare professionals seeking to understand the latest treatments, and anyone interested in the intersection of medicine and wellness.

Join me as we explore how these powerful tools can offer a new lease on life. Backed by science and proven by personal experience. Here, we begin a conversation about a revolutionary approach to weight loss that can potentially change lives, just as it changed mine. Let's start this transformative journey together.

www.kellykelswellness.com

## UNLOCKING WEIGHT LOSS:
## A Comprehensive Guide to Weight Loss Medications

Obesity has become a defining health challenge of our time. In the United States, over 40% of adults are classified as obese. It's not just about vanity. **Obesity is a Chronic Disease**, a fact recognized by the American Medical Association (AMA) in their landmark classification in 2013. Obesity is a complex disease linked to a multitude of serious health conditions, such as heart disease, type 2 diabetes, cancers, and more.

Unlocking Weight Loss: A Comprehensive Guide to Weight Loss Medications seeks to demystify the world of weight loss medications, providing you with the information and insights needed to make informed decisions about your health. This book is not a one-size-fits-all solution but a resource designed to empower you in collaboration with healthcare providers on your weight loss journey.

We will navigate the some of the most popular weight loss medications, shedding light on their mechanisms, potential benefits, and associated risks. Each medication is examined in detail, from well-known options like Orlistat and Phentermine to newer medications like Zepbound. You will have the understanding necessary for informed discussions with your healthcare provider.

Understanding obesity and its health impact is paramount. We will dive into the health risks associated with excess weight. We will provide a foundation for recognizing the importance of effective weight management. This book emphasizes the need for indivdualized solutions, encouraging you to consider weight loss medications as part of a broader approach.

## UNLOCKING WEIGHT LOSS:
## A Comprehensive Guide to Weight Loss Medications

This is not just a catalog of medications. This is a guide addressing the crucial aspect of candidacy and assessment. We will explore a brief history of weight-loss drugs, the criteria for considering them, the medical evaluations involved, and the vital role of professional guidance in making informed decisions about weight loss medications.

This book doesn't promote a magic pill mentality. Instead, it emphasizes the integration of medications with lifestyle changes. It should be understood that the role of diet, physical activity, and behavioral modifications, is foundational underscoring the necessity of a multifaceted approach for long-term success.

Let's navigate this path together, armed with knowledge, empowerment, and the tools to unlock the doors to a life of improved well-being.

## History Of Weight Loss Medications:

### 1800s-1930s: Thyroid Extracts and Laxatives

In the late 1800s and early 1900s, various unregulated potions and remedies were popular for weight loss. One of the first scientifically recognized approaches involved using thyroid hormone extracts. Thyroid hormone extracts were used in the 1890s after discovering that thyroid hormones could accelerate metabolism. Unfortunately, side effects included palpitations and high blood pressure.

### 1930s-1950s: Dinitrophenol and Amphetamines

In the 1930s, Dinitrophenol (DNP) came out. It dramatically increased metabolism but was quickly found to be extremely dangerous, causing serious side effects and even death. During World War II, amphetamines became popular as they reduced appetite and were used widely for weight loss until their addictive properties and cardiovascular risks were discovered.

### 1950s-1970s: Appetite Suppressants

The post-war era saw the FDA approval of various appetite suppressants, most notably phentermine, in 1959, which is still in use today. Another significant development was the combination drug fenfluramine/phentermine (fen-phen), which was introduced in the 1970s.

### 1980s-2000s: Fen-Phen and Its Aftermath

Fen-phen became highly popular in the 1990s. However, it was withdrawn from the market in 1997 after it was linked to heart valve disease and pulmonary hypertension. This led to a more cautious FDA approach toward approving weight loss medications.

# History Of Weight Loss Medications:

## 1800s-1930s : Thyroid Extracts and Laxatives

In the late 1800s and early 1900s, various unregulated potions and remedies were popular for weight loss. One of the first scientifically recognized approaches involved using thyroid hormone extracts. Thyroid hormone extracts were used in the 1890s after discovering that thyroid hormones could accelerate metabolism. Unfortunately, side effects included palpitations and high blood pressure.

## 1930s-1950s : Dinitrophenol and Amphetamines

In the 1930s, Dinitrophenol (DNP) came out. It dramatically increased metabolism but was quickly found to be extremely dangerous, causing serious side effects and even death. During World War II, amphetamines became popular as they reduced appetite and were used widely for weight loss until their addictive properties and cardiovascular risks were discovered.

## 1950s-1970s : Appetite Suppressants

The post-war era saw the FDA approval of various appetite suppressants, most notably phentermine, in 1959, which is still in use today. Another significant development was the combination drug fenfluramine/phentermine (fen-phen), which was introduced in the 1970s.

## 1980s-2000s : Fen-Phen and Its Aftermath

Fen-phen became highly popular in the 1990s. However, it was withdrawn from the market in 1997 after it was linked to heart valve disease and pulmonary hypertension. This led to a more cautious FDA approach toward approving weight loss medications.

## Criteria for Considering Weight Loss Medications

When deciding which weight loss medication is best for you, it is crucial to adhere to a comprehensive set of criteria to ensure both the efficacy and safety of the chosen medication. The decision to incorporate weight loss medications into a treatment plan should be made in consultation with a qualified healthcare provider, taking into account your unique health profile and needs as an individual. Several key criteria should careful be consideration:

**BMI and Health Risk Assessment:** Evaluate your Body Mass Index (BMI) and associated health risks. Weight loss medications are typically recommended for individuals with a BMI of 30 or higher or 27 or higher with obesity-related conditions. Assessing the overall health risk associated with excess weight guides the appropriateness of medication intervention.

**Failed Lifestyle Modifications:** Prioritize weight loss medications if you have been unsuccessful in achieving significant weight loss through lifestyle modifications, including diet and exercise. Medications should complement, not replace, a healthy and active lifestyle.

**Comprehensive Medical History:** Conduct a thorough examination of your medical history, including any pre-existing conditions, allergies, medications, and family history. Certain medical conditions may warn against the use of specific weight-loss medications, may require alternative approaches.

**Psychological Evaluation:** Consider the psychological factors influencing weight management. If you are struggling with emotional eating, binge eating, or other psychological issues, you may benefit from medications that address both physical and psychological aspects of weight gain.

## Criteria for Considering Weight Loss Medications
(continued)

**Patient Commitment and Compliance:** Make sure that you are committed to making the necessary lifestyle changes and are willing to adhere to the prescribed medication regimen. Being compliant is crucial to successful weight loss interventions.

**Potential Side Effects and Contraindications:** Thoroughly discuss potential side effects, contraindications, and interactions with existing medications. Your safety is paramount, and a careful risk-benefit analysis should be conducted to minimize adverse effects.

## Medical Assessment Involved in Prescribing Weight Loss Medications

Prescribing weight loss medications involves a comprehensive medical assessment to ensure the safety and efficacy of the treatment for each individual. This process typically begins with a thorough assessment of your medical history, including any pre-existing conditions, current medications, and previous weight loss attempts. The healthcare provider will also inquire about lifestyle factors, dietary habits, and physical activity levels.

A crucial aspect of the medical assessment is the determination of your body mass index (BMI), which helps classify the severity of obesity and guides the decision-making process for prescribing weight loss medications. Additionally, clinicians may assess other risk factors, such as hypertension, diabetes, and cardiovascular disease, which can influence the choice of medication.

Physical examinations are often conducted to detect any underlying health issues that may affect the patient's ability to tolerate weight loss medications. Vital signs, such as blood pressure and heart rate, are closely monitored to evaluate the overall health and cardiovascular fitness of the individual.

Laboratory tests are commonly used in medical assessments to assess baseline values and potential complications for weight-loss medications. These tests may include blood lipid profiles, liver function tests, and glucose levels. The results provide valuable information about the patient's metabolic health and aid in identifying any potential risks associated with the prescribed medications.

Psychosocial factors also play a significant role in medically evaluating weight loss medications. Healthcare providers often explore the patient's mental health, stress levels, and motivation to ensure a holistic approach to weight management. Addressing any underlying psychological or emotional factors is essential for long-term success in weight loss.

# Making Informed Decisions Before Receiving Weight Loss Medications

Making informed decisions about your health, especially when considering weight loss medications, is a crucial aspect of achieving lasting well-being. Professional guidance plays a vital role in navigating the complex landscape of weight management, ensuring that you can make choices aligned with your unique health needs and goals.

Weight loss medications, while potentially effective, are not one-size-fits-all solutions. Professional guidance from healthcare providers, such as physicians, nutritionists, and registered dietitians, is crucial when assessing your overall health, underlying conditions, and lifestyle factors. These experts have the knowledge to determine whether weight loss medications are a suitable option, taking into account factors like your existing medical conditions, medication interactions, and potential side effects.

Professional guidance extends beyond the prescription of medications. Healthcare providers give invaluable insights into comprehensive weight management strategies, including personalized nutrition plans, exercise routines, and behavioral modifications. They can help you understand the root causes of your weight concerns, addressing both physical and psychological aspects of your well-being. They educate you about the benefits and limitations of weight loss medications, ensuring that expectations are realistic and aligned with achievable outcomes.

Monitoring and follow-up are important components of professional guidance. Regular check-ins allow healthcare providers to assess the medication's effectiveness, address any emerging issues, and make necessary adjustments to your plan of care. This ongoing support helps you stay on track, fostering a collaborative and informed approach to weight management.

# Health Risks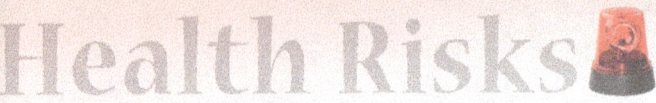

## Understanding Obesity and Its Health Risks

Overweight/Obesity is classified using the **B**ody **M**ass Index (BMI)

### What is the Body Mass Index?

BMI is a screening tool that estimates your body fat based on weight versus height. It's calculated by dividing weight in kilograms by the square of height in meters. While not a perfect measure of body fat, it's widely accepted as an indicator of health risks associated with weight.

**BMI Classifications:**
BMI is interpreted into categories, indicating potential health risks:

- Underweight: BMI below **18.5**
- Healthy weight: BMI between **18.5** and **24.9**
- Overweight: BMI between **25** and **29.9**
- Obese: BMI of **30 or higher**

**Obesity Classification:**
Obesity is further broken down to reflect varying degrees of severity:

- Class 1 Obesity: BMI of **30** to **34.9**
- Class 2 Obesity: BMI of **35** to **39.9**
- Class 3 Obesity: BMI of **40 or higher** (also referred to as severe or extreme obesity)

### How is BMI Used in Obesity Management?

**Initial Screening:** BMI is a quick and easy tool to get an initial idea of your weight status and need for further evaluation.

**Risk Assessment:** BMI helps healthcare providers understand associated health risks and determine if a more detailed body composition analysis is needed.

**Tracking Progress:** BMI can be used to monitor weight changes over time in response to interventions.

# Health Risks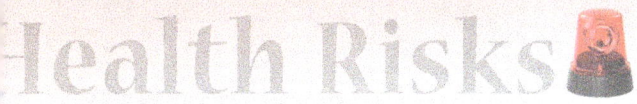

## Limitations of BMI

**BMI has some limitations to be aware of:**

- **Doesn't distinguish between fat and muscle:** Muscular individuals may have a high BMI without excess body fat.

- **May not reflect body fat distribution:** Where fat is stored (e.g., abdominal fat) carries additional health risks not reflected in BMI alone.

- **Variations across populations:** BMI doesn't properly reflect some ethnic groups and will need adjustments.

## Health Risks Associated With Obesity:

Obesity is a complex health condition that poses various health risks. It significantly increases the risk of developing several chronic diseases and health conditions including:

- **Heart Disease and Stroke:** Obesity can lead to high blood pressure, abnormal blood lipid levels, and diabetes. These factors increase the risk of heart disease and stroke.

- **Type 2 Diabetes:** Obesity is a major risk factor for type 2 diabetes, a condition where the body's blood sugar levels are too high due to insulin resistance.

- **Certain Cancers:** Obesity increases the risk of developing various types of cancer, including breast, colon, endometrium, kidney, esophagus, and pancreatic cancer.

- **Digestive Problems:** Obesity can lead to various gastrointestinal issues, including GERD (gastroesophageal reflux disease), gallstones, and liver diseases.

- **Sleep Apnea and Breathing Problems:** Excess weight can contribute to sleep apnea and other breathing problems, which interrupt sleep patterns and lead to daytime fatigue.

# Health Risks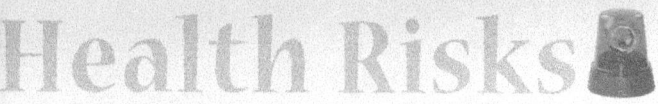

## Health Risks Associated With Obesity (continued)

- **Osteoarthritis:** Extra weight places additional pressure on joints, leading to wear and tear. This can cause osteoarthritis, particularly in the knees, hips, and lower back.

- **Gynecological and Sexual Health Issues:** Obesity can cause menstrual issues and infertility in women. In men, obesity may be associated with erectile dysfunction.

- **Mental Health Issues:** There is also a psychological aspect, as obesity can lead to mental health issues, such as depression, anxiety, and low self-esteem due to societal stigma and personal body image issues.

- **Metabolic Syndrome**: This is a group of conditions that includes high blood pressure, high blood sugar, excess body fat around the waist, and abnormal cholesterol levels, all of which increase the risk of heart disease, stroke, and diabetes.

It is important to approach obesity not just as a matter of weight but as a complex health disease requiring a multifaceted treatment approach, including lifestyle changes, medical intervention, and possibly surgery. Consulting healthcare providers for personalized advice and treatment plans is crucial for effectively managing obesity and reducing the associated health risks.

# Weight Loss Medications

## Orlistat (Xenical, Alli)

Orlistat is a medication used to treat obesity. Its main function is to inhibit the absorption of fats from your diet, thereby reducing caloric intake. Orlistat works by inhibiting the enzyme lipase, which is required for breaking down and absorbing dietary fats. As fats are not absorbed, they are excreted undigested in the feces.

### History and FDA Approval

Drugmaker Roche developed Orlistat in the late 1980s. It was approved by the U.S. Food and Drug Administration (FDA) for prescription use in 1999 under the brand name Xenical (120 mg). In 2007, the FDA approved a lower-dose, over-the-counter version of Orlistat (60 mg) under the brand name Alli.

### Mechanism of Action

Orlistat's primary mechanism is inhibiting gastric and pancreatic lipases, enzymes involved in the breakdown of dietary fats. By blocking these enzymes, Orlistat prevents the breakdown of triglycerides into absorbable free fatty acids and monoacylglycerols, thus reducing the amount of fat absorbed by the body. Orlistat's primary mechanism is inhibiting gastric and pancreatic lipases, enzymes involved in breaking down dietary fats.

# Weight Loss Medications

## Orlistat (Xenical, Alli)

### Usage
Orlistat can be used for both short-term and long-term weight management, simultaneously with a reduced-calorie diet and physical exercise. Its effectiveness for long-term use, beyond six months to a year, varies among individuals based on their adherence to lifestyle changes.

### Dosing
For prescription strength (Xenical, **120 mg**) and over-the-counter version (Alli, **60 mg**), the recommended dose is one capsule taken with each main meal containing fat (up to three capsules daily).

### Side Effects
Common side effects include gastrointestinal issues such as oily fecal spotting, flatulence with discharge, urgent bowel movements, and fatty or oily stools. These effects are generally mild and can be reduced by adhering to a low-fat diet. Serious side effects are rare but can include liver injury and kidney stones. Orlistat can block vitamins A, D, E, and K, which are fat-soluble vitamins.

### Weight Loss Potential
Studies have shown that Orlistat, combined with lifestyle changes, can lead to an average weight loss of 5-10% of initial body weight over a year. The actual amount of weight loss varies by individual. Keep in mind, Orlistat does not suppress appetite.

# Weight Loss Medications

## Orlistat (Xenical, Alli)

### Cost

The cost of Orlistat can vary widely depending on the brand (Xenical vs. Alli), dosage, and whether it's covered by insurance. Over-the-counter versions (Alli) tend to be cheaper than prescription options. Alli costs around $65/month more or less.

### Use in Children

Orlistat is approved for use in adolescents aged 12 and older. However, its use in children should be under the supervision of a healthcare provider, with careful consideration of the potential benefits and risks.

## Special Instructions:

- **Missed Dose**: If you miss a dose, take it as soon as possible unless it's been more than an hour since you ate. If it's been over an hour, skip the missed dose and resume your regular schedule.

- **Store at room temperature**, away from moisture and heat.

- **Additional Information:** Must be taken with a meal containing fat, as it blocks fat absorption. Avoid high-fat meals to reduce gastrointestinal side effects.

# Weight Loss Medications

## Phentermine (Adipex, Lomaira)

Phentermine, also known as Adipex and Lomaira (low dose), Is one of the most commonly prescribed weight loss medications in the United States.

### History and FDA Approval

Phentermine was approved by the FDA in 1959, making it one of the oldest drugs on the market used for obesity. It was initially part of a combination drug for weight loss known as fen-phen (a combination of fenfluramine and phentermine). However, fenfluramine was taken off the market in 1997, due to concerns about heart valve disease, **leaving phentermine available for individual use.**

### Mechanism of Action

Phentermine is a sympathomimetic amine that stimulates the central nervous system (nerves and brain), which increases your heart rate and blood pressure and decreases your appetite.

# Weight Loss Medications

## Phentermine (Adipex, Lomaira)

### Usage

The FDA approves Phentermine for short-term use, typically 12 weeks, as part of a plan that includes exercise, dietary changes, and behavior modification for weight loss. However, some healthcare providers prescribe Phentermine beyond 12 weeks. New studies show that it is likely to be safe. The longer Phentermine is used the greater the probability of developing tolerance, which occurs when you need a higher dose of medication to achieve the same goal.

### Dosing

Phentermine is available in several forms and strengths, including capsules and tablets. It is taken once a day before breakfast or 1 to 2 hours after breakfast. Avoid evening dosing due to the risk of insomnia. Dosing can vary based on the specific product and patient needs. Doses range from **8mg** (Lomaira), **15mg**, **30mg**, and **37.5mg**.

# Weight Loss Medications

## Phentermine (Adipex, Lomaira)

### Side Effects

Common side effects include increased heart rate, elevated blood pressure, insomnia, nervousness, dizziness, and gastrointestinal symptoms such as dry mouth and constipation. Serious side effects can include dependency, heart-related issues, and psychological effects. Individuals with a history of stroke or heart disease may not be good candidates for Phentermine. If you have glaucoma, Phentermine may increase eye pressure even more. Phentermine may also increase thyroid levels. Consult your physician to see if Phentermine is appropriate for you. Phentermine is a controlled substance and can be habit-forming.

### Weight Loss Potential

Weight loss varies by individual but is generally modest. Studies have shown an average weight loss of **5%** to **10%** of initial body weight over 12 weeks with proper diet and exercise along with phentermine use.

# Weight Loss Medications

## Phentermine (Adipex, Lomaira)

### Cost

The cost of phentermine can vary widely depending on the dosage, quantity, and whether you have insurance coverage. Generally, it is considered one of the more affordable prescription weight loss medications. Prices range from $4-$22 for a 30-day supply.

### Use in Children

Phentermine is not FDA-approved for use in children under 16. Safety and efficacy in pediatric patients have not been established.

## Special Instructions:

- **Missed Dose:** If you miss a dose, take it as soon as you remember. If it's close to your next scheduled dose, skip the missed dose. Do not take it late in the day to avoid insomnia.

- **Refrigeration Requirements:** Store at room temperature, away from heat and moisture.

- **Additional Information:** Take in the morning to prevent sleep disturbances. Avoid using other stimulant medications.

# Weight Loss Medications

## Qsymia (Phentermine/Topiramate)

Qsymia is a prescription medication that combines Phentermine and Topiramate in an extended release capsule. It is for weight loss and weight management in adults with obesity or who are overweight with weight related conditions such as high blood pressure, type 2 diabetes, or high cholesterol.

### History and FDA Approval

Qsymia was developed by Vivus Inc. and received approval from the U.S. Food and Drug Administration (FDA) on July 17, 2012. This approval marked Qsymia as one of the first new weight loss drugs to be approved by the FDA in over a decade, offering a new treatment option for millions of Americans struggling with obesity.

### Mechanism of Action

Qsymia combines two active ingredients:

**Phentermine** is an appetite suppressant that reduces appetite and helps control cravings.

**Topiramate**, originally approved as an anticonvulsant and migraine prophylaxis medication, is thought to induce weight loss through several mechanisms. These include:

- Increasing satiety (the feeling of fullness)
- Making foods taste less appealing
- Increasing calorie expenditure

# Weight Loss Medications

## Qsymia (Phentermine/Topiramate)

### Usage

Qsymia is approved for long-term use. Clinical trials supporting the approval of Qsymia demonstrated significant weight loss when taken for up to one year. This indicates its effectiveness as a long-term weight management solution when combined with diet and exercise.

### Cost

Prices vary based on dosage and location. While some insurance plans may cover it, many do not, making out-of-pocket costs a consideration for you. With various discount coupons prices vary as Qsymia has a savings coupon that can be used at the pharmacy. Qsymia also has a program called Qsymia Engage. This program offers monthly support and Qsymia home delivery.
Go to

https://qsymiaengage.com/
for more information.

### Use in Children

Qsymia is approved for use in children 12 and older with obesity.

# Weight Loss Medications

## Qsymia (Phentermine/Topiramate)

### Dosing

Qsymia is an oral medication that is available in four dosage strengths, allowing for flexibility in dosing. Treatment typically starts with a lower dose, which can be adjusted based on the patient's response and tolerance. The medication is taken once daily in the morning, with or without food, to minimize the risk of insomnia.

- The recommended starting dose is **3.75 mg/23 mg** (Phentermine 3.75mg/Topiramate 23 mg) once daily for 14 days.
- After 14 days it may be increased to **7.5 mg/46 mg** (Phentermine 7.5 mg/Topiramate 46 mg)
- After 12 weeks of treatment with Qsymia **7.5 mg/46 mg**, weight loss should be evaluated. If you or a child (12 or older) has not lost at least 3% of your starting body weight, then the dose can be increased to Qsymia **11.5mg/69mg** ( Phentermine 11.5 mg/Topiramate 69 mg) daily for 14 days.
- After 14 days, Qsymia is increased to (Phentermine 15 mg/Topiramate 92 mg).
- After 12 weeks of Qsymia **15 mg/96 mg** (Phentermine 15 mg/Topiramate 96 mg), if you or a child has not lost at least 5% of starting weight, Qsymia may be discontinued because meaningful weight loss has not been achieved.

The dosages mentioned are general guidelines. Your doctor will recommend dosing based on your individual needs. Discontinuation of Qsymia should be gradual. **Qsymia 15 mg/96 mg** (Phentermine 15mg/Topiramate 96mg) should be taken once daily every other day for at least one week. **Stopping Qsymia suddenly can cause seizures.**

# Weight Loss Medications

## Qsymia (Phentermine/Topiramate)

### Side Effects

Common side effects of Qsymia include tingling in the hands and feet, dizziness, altered taste sensation, insomnia, constipation, and dry mouth. More serious side effects may include increased heart rate, suicidal thoughts or actions, and eye problems like glaucoma. It also carries a risk for birth defects if taken by pregnant women, necessitating effective birth control for women of childbearing age who use the medication. Individuals with end-stage renal disease or dialysis should avoid using Qsymia. If suicidal thoughts occur, call your healthcare provider immediately.

### Weight Loss Potential

Clinical trials have shown that by taking Qsymia, you can achieve significant weight loss, with an average loss of 6.7% to 8.9% of body weight, depending on the dose, over one year when combined with a reduced-calorie diet and regular exercise.

## Special Instructions:

- **Missed Dose:** If you miss a dose, skip it and resume your regular schedule. Do not double the dose to make up for a missed one.
- **Refrigeration Requirements:** No refrigeration required; store at room temperature.
- **Additional Information:** Take once daily in the morning to reduce the risk of insomnia. Ensure adequate fluid intake to prevent kidney stones.

# Weight Loss Medications

## Contrave (Naltrexone/Bupropion)

Contrave (Naltrexone/Bupropion) is a prescription weight-loss medication that combines two drugs, Naltrexone 8 mg and Bupropion 90 mg, in an extended-release tablet. It is used for weight management in adults with a body mass index (BMI) of 30 or greater (obese) or 27 or greater (overweight) who have at least one weight-related condition, such as high blood pressure, type 2 diabetes, or high cholesterol. Contrave is an opioid antagonist, meaning it blocks the effects of opioid drugs.

### History and FDA Approval

Contrave was developed by Orexigen Therapeutics and received approval from the U.S. Food and Drug Administration (FDA) on September 10, 2014. The approval came after the FDA had initially rejected the drug in 2011, requesting further studies to assess its cardiovascular risk profile. Following additional studies, the FDA concluded that Contrave's benefits outweigh its potential risks when used for weight management in specific patient populations.

### Mechanism of Action

Contrave's mechanism of action for weight loss is not entirely understood but is believed to involve the combined effects of its two components:

- **Naltrexone,** primarily used for the treatment of alcohol and opioid dependence, is thought to block the effects of beta-endorphin and other endogenous opioids on the reward circuit, reducing food cravings.
- **Bupropion,** an antidepressant and smoking cessation aid, is believed to act on the central nervous system to increase dopamine and norepinephrine levels, which help in controlling appetite and energy expenditure.

The combination of these two drugs affects the brain's reward and control centers, which regulate appetite and food cravings.

# Weight Loss Medications

## Contrave (Naltrexone/Bupropion)

### Usage
Contrave is intended for long-term use in weight management, alongside a reduced-calorie diet and increased physical activity. Clinical trial data has supported its effectiveness in maintaining weight loss and safety for long-term use beyond one year.

### Dosing
Contrave is taken orally, typically starting with:

- Week 1 - **1 tablet** in the morning
- Week 2 - **2 tablets**, one tablet in the morning and one tablet in the evening
- Week 3 - **3 tablets**, two tablets in the morning and one tablet in the evening
- Week 4 and onward - **4 tablets**, two tablets in the morning and two tablets in the evening

### Side Effects
Common side effects include nausea, constipation, headache, vomiting, dizziness, insomnia, dry mouth, and diarrhea. Serious side effects may include seizures, increased blood pressure, liver damage, and the risk of suicidal thoughts and behavior, which are more associated with bupropion.

### Weight Loss Potential
Clinical trials have shown that adults taking Contrave, along with diet and exercise, lost more weight compared to those who were on diet and exercise alone. On average, you can expect to lose **5%** to **10%** of your body weight over a year with proper lifestyle changes.

# Weight Loss Medications

## Contrave (Naltrexone/Bupropion)

### Cost

The cost of Contrave can be relatively high, as it is a brand-name drug without a generic equivalent available. Prices vary, and while some insurance plans may cover it, many do not. Patient assistance programs may be available to help reduce the cost. Go to www.contrave.com for information on their prescription program.

### Use in Children

Contrave is not approved for use in people under 18. Safety and efficacy have not been established in pediatric patients.

## Special Instructions:

- **Missed Dose:** Skip the missed dose and take the next dose at the regular time. **Do not double up on doses.**

- **Refrigeration Requirements:** Store at room temperature, away from heat and moisture.

- **Additional Information:** Take it with food, but avoid taking it too close to bedtime due to potential insomnia.

# Weight Loss Medications

## Saxenda (Liraglutide)

Saxenda (Liraglutide) is a prescription medication used for weight management simultaneously with a reduced-calorie diet and increased physical activity. It is intended for adults with a body mass index (BMI) of 30 kg or higher (obese) or 27 kg or higher (overweight) in the presence of at least one weight-related comorbidity condition such as high blood pressure, type 2 diabetes, or dyslipidemia, and for children aged 12 years and older who weigh more than 60 kg (132 lbs) with certain conditions.

### History and FDA Approval

Saxenda is developed by Novo Nordisk, a global healthcare company with a significant presence in the diabetes care market. Liraglutide, the active ingredient in Saxenda, was first approved by the FDA in 2010 under the brand name Victoza to treat type 2 diabetes. Later, after additional studies demonstrated its efficacy in weight management, the FDA approved Saxenda specifically for weight management in December 2014.

### Mechanism of Action

Saxenda works by mimicking the hormone GLP-1 (glucagon-like peptide-1) that is naturally produced in the intestines. GLP-1 is released after eating and stimulates insulin secretion, which helps lower blood sugar levels. Additionally, GLP-1 reduces appetite and food intake and slows gastric emptying by acting on the central nervous system, which contributes to weight loss.

# Weight Loss Medications

## Saxenda (Liraglutide)

### Usage
Saxenda is for long-term use. Clinical trials supporting its approval have shown significant weight loss when used over an extended period, alongside a low-calorie diet and increased physical activity.

### Dosing
Saxenda is administered daily via subcutaneous injection and comes in a single pen that requires a daily needle change. You dial the pen to the desired dose. The pen can be used for 30 days, then must be discarded. The dosing starts at 0.6 mg per day and is increased weekly over five weeks to the recommended daily dose of 3.0 mg. This gradual increase helps minimize gastrointestinal side effects.

- Week 1 - **0.6 mg**
- Week 2 - **1.2 mg**
- Week 3 - **1.8 mg**
- Week 4 - **2.4 mg**
- Week 5 - **3.0 mg** max

### Side Effects
Common side effects of Saxenda include nausea, vomiting, diarrhea, constipation, and abdominal pain. Serious side effects can include pancreatitis, gallbladder disease, renal impairment, and increased heart rate. There is also a risk of thyroid C-cell tumors, as seen in animal studies, although it's not clear if this applies to humans.

### Weight Loss Potential
Clinical trials show that people using Saxenda, combined with diet and exercise, can expect to lose **5%** to **10%** of their starting body weight over a year. However, individual results can vary.

# Weight Loss Medications

## Saxenda (Liraglutide)

### Cost

With an approximate cost of $1400/month, Saxenda is one of the more expensive weight management medications on the market. The cost can vary significantly depending on location, insurance coverage, and pharmacy pricing. You may be eligible for savings cards or patient assistance programs offered by Novo Nordisk.

### Use in Children

In June 2019, the FDA approved Saxenda for use in youth aged 12 years and older who weigh more than 60 kg (132 lbs) with certain conditions. This approval was based on a study showing that Saxenda helped adolescents lose weight effectively.

### Special Instructions:

- **Missed Dose:** If a dose is missed, skip it and resume the next dose at the regular time. Do not take an extra dose.
- **Refrigeration Requirements:** Refrigerate until use. Once opened, it can be kept at room temperature for up to 30 days.
- **Additional Information:** Inject subcutaneously, rotating the injection site each time to prevent irritation.

For more information on Saxenda, visit their website at www.saxenda.com.

# Weight Loss Medications

## Wegovy (Semaglutide)

Wegovy (Semaglutide) is an injectable prescription medication used for chronic weight management. It belongs to a class of drugs known as GLP-1 receptor agonists, similar to liraglutide (Saxenda), but with a longer duration of action that allows for weekly administration. Wegovy is indicated for use in adults with obesity (body mass index [BMI] of 30 kg or greater) or overweight (BMI of 27 kg or greater) with at least one weight-related comorbidity such as hypertension, type 2 diabetes mellitus or dyslipidemia, in addition to a reduced-calorie diet and increased physical activity. Here's an overview of Wegovy:

### History and FDA Approval

Wegovy, developed by Novo Nordisk, is a higher dose of the drug semaglutide, which is also used at lower doses under the brand name Ozempic for treating type 2 diabetes. The U.S. Food and Drug Administration (FDA) approved Wegovy for weight management in June 2021, making it one of the latest additions to the arsenal of medications for obesity.

### Mechanism of Action

Semaglutide, the active ingredient in Wegovy, is a GLP-1 (glucagon-like peptide-1) receptor agonist. It mimics the action of the GLP-1 hormone, which is involved in regulating appetite and food intake. By activating GLP-1 receptors, semaglutide increases insulin secretion decreases glucagon secretion, and slows gastric emptying. This combination of effects contributes to reduced appetite and caloric intake, leading to weight loss.

# Weight Loss Medications

## Wegovy (Semaglutide)

### Usage

Wegovy is for long-term use in chronic weight management. It is not specified for short-term weight loss but rather as part of a comprehensive weight management program that includes dietary changes and increased physical activity.

### Dosing

Wegovy is administered once weekly via subcutaneous injection. Wegovy comes in single-use pens that are discarded after each use. The dosing regimen starts at 0.25 mg per week and is gradually increased over several weeks to the recommended maintenance dose of 2.4 mg per week to improve gastrointestinal tolerability.

1 Shot Weekly
- Month 1 - **0.25 mg**
- Month 2 - **0.50 mg**
- Month 3 - **1 mg**
- Month 4 - **1.7 mg**
- Month 5 - **2.4 mg** max

# Weight Loss Medications

## Wegovy (Semaglutide)

### Side Effects

Common side effects of Wegovy include nausea, vomiting, diarrhea, stomach pain, and constipation. These side effects are generally mild to moderate in severity and tend to diminish over time. More serious side effects can include pancreatitis, gallbladder problems, kidney problems, and a possible increased risk of certain thyroid tumors.

### Weight Loss Potential

Clinical trials have shown that Wegovy can cause significant weight loss. Participants in these trials lost an average of 10-15% of their body weight over 68 weeks when combined with a reduced-calorie diet and increased physical activity. The exact amount of weight loss can vary depending on individual factors, including diet and exercise adherence.

# Weight Loss Medications

## Wegovy (Semaglutide)

### Cost

Wegovy is one of the more expensive weight management medications, with costs that can be prohibitive for some patients. The cost can start at $1300 and up. Insurance coverage for Wegovy varies, and some patients may be eligible for manufacturer-sponsored savings programs or assistance.

Visit www.wegovy.com for further information.

### Use in Children

Wegovy was not approved for pediatric patients. However, given the evolving nature of pharmaceutical approvals and indications, it's important to consult current resources or a healthcare provider for the most up-to-date information regarding its use in children.

# Weight Loss Medications

## Wegovy (Semaglutide)

### Special Instructions:

**Missed Dose:**
- If you miss a dose and it has been less than 5 days since the missed dose, take it as soon as possible.
- If more than 5 days have passed, skip the missed dose and take the next dose at the regular time.

**Refrigeration Requirements:**
- Store in the refrigerator before use.
- After first use, Wegovy can be kept at room temperature (up to 86°F) for up to 28 days.
- Do not freeze Wegovy, and protect it from light.

**Additional Information:**
- Inject subcutaneously, rotating the injection site each time to prevent irritation.

**As of March 2024, the FDA approved Wegovy for heart disease prevention usage.**

# Weight Loss Medications

## Zepbound (Tirzepatide)

Zepbound Tirzepatide is an injectable prescription used in chronic weight management. Eli Lilly and Company developed it. By adding this extra GIP component, it builds upon the success of other GLP-1 receptor agonists like Semaglutide.

### History and FDA Approval

Tirzepatide belongs to a newer class of diabetes and weight-loss drugs known as incretin mimetics. These drugs mimic the effects of hormones called incretins that help regulate blood sugar and appetite. Type 2 Diabetes (Mounjaro): Tirzepatide's initial FDA approval in May 2022 was for the brand name Mounjaro, indicated as a treatment for adults with type 2 diabetes. (Zepbound): In November 2023, the FDA approved Tirzepatide for chronic weight management under the brand name Zepbound. It was approved for use in adults with obesity (BMI of 30 or greater) or those who are overweight (BMI of 27 or greater) and also have at least one other weight-related health condition (like high blood pressure, type 2 diabetes, or high cholesterol).

- GIP and GLP-1: Tirzepatide is a unique dual agonist. It activates receptors for two important incretins.

- Glucagon-like Peptide-1 (GLP-1): GLP-1 plays a significant role in blood glucose control, stimulating insulin release, and slowing gastric emptying (making you feel full), and reducing appetite. Glucose-dependent Insulinotropic Polypeptide (GIP): GIP primarily aids in insulin secretion after food intake and impacts fat metabolism.

Eli Lilly and Company developed Tirzepatide. By adding this extra GIP component, it builds upon the success of other GLP-1 receptor agonists, like semaglutide.

# Weight Loss Medications

## Zepbound (Tirzepatide)

### Mechanism of Action

Dosage is gradually titrated over several weeks, starting at a low dose (2.5mg) and incrementally increasing to reduce potential side effects.

- Tirzepatide's actions on both GLP-1 and GIP receptors lead to several effects beneficial for weight loss:

- Reduced Appetite and Food Intake: Increased feelings of fullness and satiety.

- Regulation of Blood Sugar: Aids in glucose control and can reduce insulin resistance.

- Improved Metabolism: Potential impact on fat burning and energy expenditure.

Studies have demonstrated impressive weight loss with Tirzepatide. Trial participants often achieved substantial weight reductions, exceeding results seen with other anti-obesity medications.

# Weight Loss Medications

## Zepbound (Tirzepatide)

### Usage

Tirzepatide comes as a once-weekly subcutaneous injection (under the skin). Zepbound is for long-term use and as part of a comprehensive weight management program that includes dietary changes and increased physical activity.

### Dosing

Zepbound is administered once weekly via subcutaneous injection. Zepbound comes in a box of 4 single-use pens. One pen is used weekly. Each set of pens (4) comes in either 2.5 mg, 5 mg, 10 mg, 12.5 mg, or 15 mg. Zepbound dosing is gradually increased over several weeks to the recommended maintenance dose of 15 mg.

1 Shot Weekly

- Month 1 - **2.5 mg**
- Month 2 - **5 mg**
- Month 3 - **7.5 mg**
- Month 4 - **10 mg**
- Month 5 - **12.5 mg**
- Month 6 - **15 mg** max

This dosing schedule may vary based on your physician's recommendation.

# Weight Loss Medications

## Zepbound (Tirzepatide)

### Side Effects

Common side effects include nausea, diarrhea, decreased appetite, vomiting, constipation, indigestion, sulfur burps, and abdominal pain. Most side effects are gastrointestinal and tend to decrease over time. More severe side effects (all although rare) include severe allergic reactions, thyroid cancer, pancreatitis, suicidal thoughts or behavior, gallbladder stones, and kidney issues, just to name a few.

### Weight Loss Potential

Clinical trials have shown significant weight loss in type 2 diabetes participants and those without diabetes. The amount of weight loss varies depending on the dose and individual factors but can be substantial, especially at higher doses. Individuals taking the highest dose of Zepbound lost approximately **21%** of their body weight over 72 weeks.

# Weight Loss Medications

## Zepbound (Tirzepatide)

### Cost

The cost of Zepbound can be quite expensive, often exceeding several hundred dollars per month. Depending on your location, look to pay $1100 and up. The exact cost can vary based on insurance coverage, pharmacy location, and whether patient assistance programs are available. Individuals with commercial insurance may be eligible for a Zepbound savings coupon. Visit www.zepbound.lilly.com

### Use in Children

As of my last update in April 2023, Zepbound was not approved for use in children. Clinical trials and studies in pediatric populations are necessary to establish safety, efficacy, and dosing guidelines for individuals under 18 years of age.

# Weight Loss Medications

## Zepbound (Tirzepatide)

### Special Instructions:

**Missed Dose:**
- If you miss a dose, take it as soon as possible within 4 days (96 hours) of the missed dose.
- If more than 4 days have passed, skip the missed dose and take the next dose at the regular time.
- The day of the weekly injection can be changed, if necessary, as long as the time between doses is at least 3 days or 72 hours.

**Refrigeration Requirements:**
- Store Zepbound in the refrigerator.
- Zepbound can be kept at room temperature (up to 86°F) for up to 21 days.
- Avoid freezing. If freezing occurs, discard the medication. Keep it away from direct light.

**Additional Information:**
- Inject subcutaneously, rotating the injection site each time to prevent irritation.

# Weight Loss Medications

| | Orlistat | Phentermine/ Topiramate ER | Naltrexone ER/ Bupropion ER | Liraglutide | Semaglutide | Tirzepatide |
|---|---|---|---|---|---|---|
| **ANTI-OBESITY PHARMACOTHERAPY IMPROVES RISK FACTORS AND COMORBIDITIES*** | | | | | | |
| Waist Circumference | ↓ | ↓ | ↓ | ↓ | ↓ | ↓ |
| Blood Pressure | ↓ | ↓ | ↑ | ↓ | ↓ | ↓ |
| Heart Rate | ↓ | — | ↑ | ↑ | ↑ | ↓ |
| LDL-C | ↓ | ↓ | ↓ | ↓ | ↓ | ↓ |
| LDL-C | ↑ | ↑ | ↑ | ↑ | ↑ | ↑ |
| Triglycerides | ↓↓ | ↓↓ | ↓↓ | ↓↓ | ↓↓ | ↓↓ |
| A1C | ↓ | ↓ | ↓ | ↓↓↓ | ↓↓↓ | ↓↓↓ |

*COMORBIDITIES : HAVING MORE THAN ONE DISEASE OR CONIDITION AT THE SAME TIME

# Common Side Effects

## Common Side Effects of Weight Loss Medication

Weight loss medications have the potential to be a valuable tool for those struggling with obesity or excess weight. However, it's important to be aware that these medications often come with side effects. Side effects range from mild to severe. Understanding common side effects and learning effective management strategies is crucial to optimizing your medication experience and reducing the likelihood of discontinuing treatment.

## Digestive Side Effects

Common digestive issues include nausea, vomiting, diarrhea, constipation, and abdominal discomfort.

## Nausea and Vomiting

- **Smaller, frequent meals:** Instead of three large meals, try eating five or six smaller portions throughout the day. This puts less stress on your digestive system.

- **Bland foods:** When nausea strikes, stick to easy-to-digest foods like crackers, plain toast, rice, bananas, and applesauce (BRAT diet). Avoid greasy, spicy, or overly sweet foods.

- **Ginger:** Ginger has natural anti-nausea properties. Try ginger tea, ginger chews, or adding fresh ginger to food.

- **Hydration:** Sip on water, clear broths, or electrolyte drinks to prevent dehydration if vomiting occurs.

- **Alcohol:** Place rubbing alcohol on a cloth and fan past your nose.

- **Over-the-counter options:** Ask your doctor if over-the-counter anti-nausea medications are an option.

## Digestive Side Effects (continued)

### Diarrhea

- **Plenty of fluids:** Dehydration is a major concern with diarrhea. Focus on water, clear broths, and electrolyte replacement drinks.
- **Modify your diet:** Temporarily limit dairy, high-fiber foods (raw vegetables, beans), caffeine, and alcohol, as these can worsen diarrhea.
- **Consult your doctor:** Let them know if diarrhea is severe or lasts for an extended period. Over-the-counter anti-diarrheal medications might be helpful, but discuss this with your doctor first.

### Constipation

- **High-fiber foods:** Gradually increase your intake of fruits, vegetables, wholegrains, and legumes. Aim for 25 to 35 grams of fiber daily.
- **Hydration is key:** Water helps soften stool and ease its passage.
- **Physical activity:** Regular exercise stimulates bowel movements.
- **Stool softeners or gentle laxatives:** If lifestyle changes don't help, discuss these options with your doctor.
- **Castor oil packs or soak a cotton ball with castor oil:** Place a soaked cotton ball in the belly button, secure with band aid or skin friendly adhesive tape. Leave it overnight or a few hours during the day.

# Common Side Effects

## Digestive Side Effects (continued)

### Abdominal Discomfort

- **Identify triggers:** Certain foods may trigger bloating and cramping. Keep a food diary to track any sensitivities.
- **Over-the-counter gas remedies:** Medications containing simethicone, such as Alka-seltzer, Gas-X, Maalox Anti-gas, and Mylanta, can help break up gas bubbles.
- **Peppermint or fennel tea:** These herbs have calming effects on the digestive system.
- **Probiotics:** Talk to your doctor about whether probiotic supplements might help restore a healthy gut-bacterial balance.
- **Inform your healthcare provider** as prescription medication may be needed.

## Digestive Side Effects (continued)

### Abdominal Discomfort

- **Identify triggers:** Certain foods may trigger bloating and cramping. Keep a food diary to track any sensitivities.
- **Over-the-counter gas remedies:** Medications containing simethicone, such as Alka-seltzer, Gas-X, Maalox Anti-gas, and Mylanta, can help break up gas bubbles.
- **Peppermint or fennel tea:** These herbs have calming effects on the digestive system.
- **Probiotics:** Talk to your doctor about whether probiotic supplements might help restore a healthy gut-bacterial balance.
- **Inform your healthcare provider** as prescription medication may be needed.

# Common ⚠ Side Effects

## Nervous System Side Effects

Common nervous system side effects include Headaches, dizziness, insomnia, restlessness, and anxiety.

### Headaches

- **Hydrate:** Dehydration is a common trigger for headaches. Make sure you're drinking plenty of water throughout the day.
- **Over-the-counter pain relievers:** Acetaminophen or ibuprofen can help with occasional headaches. Consult your doctor before regular use.
- **Relaxation techniques:** Stress can worsen headaches. Try mindfulness, deep breathing exercises, or gentle yoga.
- **Caffeine moderation:** Monitor your caffeine intake, as both excessive amounts and sudden withdrawal can cause headaches.

### Dizziness

- **Sit or lie down immediately:** This prevents falls if you feel faint.
- **Slow movements:** Get up slowly from seated or lying positions to allow your blood pressure to adjust.
- **Hydration and light snacks:** Dehydration and low blood sugar can contribute to dizziness. Small, frequent snacks and adequate fluid intake may help.
- **Consult your doctor:** Persistent dizziness may require medication adjustments or further evaluation.

## Common ⚠ Side Effects

### Nervous System Side Effects (continued)

#### Insomnia and Restlessness

- **Medication timing:** If possible, take your medication earlier in the day to minimize its impact on sleep.
- **Consistent sleep schedule:** Maintain a regular bedtime and wake-up time, even on weekends.
- **Relaxing bedtime routine:** Wind down with a warm bath, calming music, or reading before bed. Avoid screens at least an hour before sleep.
- **Avoid stimulants:** Limit caffeine and nicotine, especially later in the day.
- **See your doctor:** If sleep issues are severe, your doctor might recommend temporary sleep aids or adjust your medication.

#### Anxiety

- **Mindfulness and relaxation techniques:** Deep breathing, meditation, and yoga can help manage anxiety.
- **Regular exercise:** Physical activity is a great way to combat stress and promote better sleep.
- **Therapy:** Talk therapy, such as cognitive behavioral therapy (CBT), can provide techniques for managing anxiety and coping with medication side effects.
- **Communicate with your doctor:** You may require added anti-anxiety medication as well.

# Common ⚠️ Side Effects

## Cardiovascular Side Effects
Cardiovascular side effects include increased heart rate and elevated blood pressure.

### Management Strategies
- **Pre-treatment Screening:** Before starting weight loss medication, your doctor will likely assess your cardiovascular health. This might include blood pressure checks, an EKG (electrocardiogram), and discussing your medical history.

- **Regular Monitoring:** Your doctor will closely monitor your heart rate and blood pressure throughout your treatment, especially at the beginning and during any dosage changes.

- **Medication Adjustments:** If you experience elevated heart rate or blood pressure, your doctor may adjust the dosage, switch to a different medication, or prescribe medications specifically to manage blood pressure.

- **Addressing Underlying Conditions:** If you have any existing heart conditions, your doctor will carefully manage them along with your weight loss treatment plan.

- **Lifestyle Choices Matter:** Maintain a heart-healthy diet, exercise regularly, manage stress, and get enough sleep. These lifestyle factors are crucial for overall cardiovascular health.

### Important Considerations
- **Individualized Approach:** The best management strategy depends on your specific medication, individual health profile, and the severity of side effects.

- **Don't Ignore Symptoms:** Report any chest pain, shortness of breath, palpitations, or other concerning cardiovascular symptoms to your doctor immediately.

- **Medication Choice:** Your doctor will carefully select a weight loss medication considering your cardiovascular risk factors and any existing conditions. Some medications may be more suitable than others for individuals with heart concerns.

# Common Side Effects

### Cardiovascular Side Effects (continued)
**Additional Tips**

- **Know Your Numbers:** Regularly check your blood pressure at home if advised by your doctor.

- **Limit Sodium:** A high-sodium diet can contribute to elevated blood pressure.

- **Manage Stress:** Stress hormones can affect your heart rate and blood pressure. Find healthy stress-management techniques.

# Common Side Effects

## Dry Mouth Side Effect

### Strategies for Relief

- **Hydrate, hydrate, hydrate:** Sip water frequently throughout the day. Carry a water bottle with you to ensure you have access at all times.
- **Stimulate saliva production:**
  - Chew sugar-free gum containing xylitol (this sweetener also helps combat tooth decay).
  - Suck on sugar-free hard candies (citrus, mint, or cinnamon flavors can be particularly stimulating).
- **Over-the-counter aids:**
  - Saliva substitutes: These sprays or rinses can temporarily moisten the mouth.
  - Mouthwashes designed for dry mouth: Look for alcohol-free options with ingredients like xylitol.
- **Humidifier:** Consider using a humidifier at night, especially during dry seasons, to add moisture to the air.
- **Avoid irritants:**
  - Limit caffeine and alcohol, as they further dehydrate you.
  - Smoking and chewing tobacco worsen dry mouth. Overly spicy or salty foods can be irritating.
  - Overly spicy or salty foods can be irritating.
- **Lip balm:** Keep your lips moisturized to prevent cracking and discomfort.

## Dry Mouth Side Effect (continued)

### Focus on Oral Health

- **Meticulous dental hygiene:** Dry mouth increases your risk for cavities and dental problems. Brush twice daily, floss regularly, and see your dentist for checkups at least twice a year.

- **Fluoride treatments:** Ask your dentist about additional fluoride rinses or gels to strengthen your teeth.

### When to See Your Doctor

- **Persistent discomfort:** If over-the-counter measures don't provide enough relief, consult your doctor for alternative treatment options.

- **Signs of infection:** See your doctor or dentist if you experience sores, white patches, or persistent bad breath, as these could signal an oral infection.

### Additional Considerations

- **Medication review:** Your doctor may be able to adjust your medication or switch to one with fewer drying side effects.

- **Underlying conditions:** Sometimes, dry mouth can be a sign of an underlying health condition like Sjögren's syndrome. If dry mouth is severe, discuss this with your doctor.

# Common Side Effects

## Fatigue, Mood Changes, and Changes in Taste

### Managing Fatigue

- **Talk to your doctor:** Discuss the severity of your fatigue, as they might want to check for underlying causes like anemia or medication interactions. Dosage adjustments or medication changes might help.
- **Prioritize sleep:** Aim for 7-8 hours of quality sleep each night. Establish a good sleep routine, keep your bedroom cool and dark, and avoid screens before bed.
- **Strategic naps:** A short nap (20-30 minutes) during the day can provide a temporary energy boost.
- **Regular exercise:** While fatigue might make this seem counterintuitive, regular physical activity can improve energy levels over time. Start with short sessions and gradually increase duration and intensity.
- **Healthy diet:** Focus on nutrient-dense foods for sustained energy, and avoid excessive sugar and processed foods that can cause energy crashes.

# Common ⚠ Side Effects

## Fatigue, Mood Changes, and Changes in Taste
(continued)

### Managing Mood Changes

- **Track your moods:** Keep a mood diary or use a mood-tracking app to identify any patterns linked to your medication schedule. This helps you and your doctor determine if the changes are related to your medication.

- **Stress management:** Techniques like meditation, yoga, or deep breathing can help manage stress and anxiety, which often worsen mood issues.

- **Exercise:** Physical activity is a natural mood booster. Aim for at least 30 minutes of moderate-intensity exercise most days of the week.

- **Therapy:** Talk therapy, like cognitive-behavioral therapy (CBT), can teach you coping mechanisms and help you reframe negative thoughts.

- **Communicate with your doctor:** Discuss the severity of any mood changes with your doctor. They might suggest medication adjustments, a switch to a different medication, or a combination of medication and therapy.

### Managing Changes in Taste

- **Experiment with flavors:** Play with different spices and herbs to find new ways to make food appealing.

- **Focus on texture:** If taste is altered, pay attention to textures. Varying crunchy, soft, or creamy foods can help with meal satisfaction.

- **Rinse often:** Use mouthwash or a saltwater rinse before meals to help neutralize any unpleasant tastes.

# Common ⚠ Side Effects

## Why is Hair Loss Happening?

- **Rapid Weight Loss:** Significant or rapid weight loss can trigger hair loss, often due to a condition called telogen effluvium. When the body undergoes rapid changes, such as substantial weight loss, it can cause more hair follicles to enter the resting (telogen) phase of the hair growth cycle, leading to increased shedding.

- **Nutritional Deficiencies:** Restrictive diets or rapid weight loss can lead to deficiencies in essential nutrients like protein, iron, zinc, biotin, and other vitamins that are crucial for hair health. GLP-1/GIP medications often suppress appetite, which might cause a reduced intake of these nutrients.

- **Hormonal Changes:** Weight loss can also cause changes in hormone levels, including those that influence hair growth. These hormonal shifts may contribute to hair thinning or loss.

- **Stress:** Both the physical stress of weight loss and the emotional stress of undergoing a significant lifestyle change can contribute to hair loss.

## What Should You Do For Hair Loss?

- **Ensure Nutritional Adequacy:**

  **Balanced Diet:** Focus on a well-balanced diet rich in proteins, vitamins (especially B vitamins), iron, zinc, and omega-3 fatty acids. Consider incorporating foods like eggs, nuts, leafy greens, and lean meats.

  **Supplements:** If your diet might be lacking, consider taking supplements like biotin, zinc, or a multivitamin after consulting with a healthcare provider.

- **Manage the Rate of Weight Loss:**

  If the weight loss is too rapid, consider slowing down the process. A steady, gradual weight loss is less likely to trigger hair loss. Work with your healthcare provider or nutritionist to develop a plan tailored to your specific needs.

- **Consult with a Healthcare Provider:**

  **Blood Tests:** Get blood work done to check for deficiencies in iron, thyroid function, or other relevant nutrients.

  **Medication Review:** Discuss with your healthcare provider whether the medication dosage needs adjustment or if additional supplements are necessary.

- **Reduce Stress:**

  Engage in stress-reducing activities like yoga, meditation, or light exercise, which can help minimize hair loss.

- **Topical Treatments:**

  Consider using over-the-counter topical treatments like minoxidil, which can help promote hair regrowth.

Addressing hair loss as soon as possible can help prevent further shedding and support healthy hair growth as you continue your weight loss journey.

# Common ⚠️ Side Effects

## Feeling Cold

Feeling cold while on GLP-1 & GLP-1/GIP medications can happen for several reasons, often related to its effects on metabolism, weight loss, and overall physiological changes. Here's a breakdown:

- **Reduced Insulation Due to Weight Loss**

    **Reason:** Semaglutide often leads to significant weight loss, which may reduce fat stores. Fat acts as an insulator, helping to maintain body temperature.

    **Result:** Less fat can make you more sensitive to cold.

- **Lowered Basal Metabolic Rate**

    **Reason:** As you lose weight, your Basal Metabolic Rate (BMR) may decrease. A lower BMR means your body produces less heat at rest.

    **Result:** You might feel colder even in normal temperatures.

- **Changes in Circulation**

    **Reason:** Weight loss and medication effects can alter blood flow. The body may prioritize blood flow to vital organs, leaving extremities like hands and feet feeling colder.

    **Result:** Increased sensitivity to cold, particularly in your limbs.

- **Impact on Appetite and Calorie Intake**

    **Reason:** Semaglutide reduces appetite, which may result in lower food intake and, consequently, less energy for heat production.

    **Result:** Feeling colder due to reduced caloric energy.

- **Hormonal Changes**

    **Reason:** GLP-1 receptor agonists like semaglutide affect gut hormones and may influence the hypothalamus, which regulates body temperature.

    **Result:** Subtle shifts in temperature regulation could cause feelings of coldness.

## Tips to Manage Feeling Cold:

- **Stay Warm:** Dress in layers, and use heated blankets or warm beverages to stay comfortable.

- **Monitor Food Intake:** Ensure you're consuming enough calories and nutrients to support metabolism and energy.

- **Hydrate:** Dehydration can exacerbate the feeling of cold.

- **Exercise:** Regular physical activity helps boost circulation and heat production.

- **Consult Your Healthcare Provider:** If the feeling of cold persists or worsens, discuss it with your doctor to rule out other causes, such as hypothyroidism or anemia.

This side effect often goes away over time as your body adjusts to the medication.

# Common Side Effects

**Common Positive**
**Side Effects of Weight Loss Medication**

**Food Noise**

Many individuals on Contrave, Saxenda, Wegovy, and Zepbound report experiencing "food noise" reduction or elimination.

> ***Food noise** refers to the constant thoughts and preoccupations around food. This includes thinking about what to eat, when to eat, how much to eat, and even if you are not hungry.*

These medications work by regulating appetite, reducing cravings, and making you feel fuller and more satisfied with smaller portions. This results in experiencing less mental preoccupation with food, reducing food noise. Individuals report feeling a new sense of freedom and are just as valuable as weight loss.

# Medications Written Off-Label for Weight Loss

Prescribing medications "off label" means using them for a purpose different from those approved by regulatory agencies like the U.S. Food and Drug Administration (FDA). Off-label prescribing is common in many areas of medicine, including weight loss. However, it's important to note that the effectiveness and safety of using these medications for weight loss may not have been fully established. Therefore, they should only be used under the guidance of a healthcare provider. Here is a list of popular medications that have been used off-label for weight loss:

- **Metformin:** Originally used to treat type 2 diabetes, it can help with weight loss in some individuals by improving insulin sensitivity and reducing hunger.

- **Topiramate:** A drug for epilepsy and migraine prevention. It can also help with weight loss by decreasing appetite and increasing feelings of fullness.

- **Bupropion:** An antidepressant that can aid weight loss by reducing appetite. It's sometimes combined with Naltrexone (a medication used for addiction treatment) in a medication specifically approved for weight loss called Contrave.

- **Zonisamide:** Another anticonvulsant drug that can have weight loss as a side effect, potentially through appetite suppression and increased energy expenditure.

- **Off-label use of ADHD medications:** Stimulant medications, such as amphetamine salts (Adderall) and methylphenidate (Ritalin), are sometimes used off-label for their appetite-suppressing effects.

## Medications Written Off Label for Weight Loss
(continued)

- **Fluoxetine:** An antidepressant that can lead to weight loss in some patients, especially in the early months of treatment.

- **Off label use of Diabetic medications:** Mounjaro, Ozempic, Rybelsus, Trulicity, Byetta, and Victoza; in many instances, these medications require Prior Authorization (PA) from your insurance company, permitting to use these medications for the purpose indicated by your healthcare provider. Generally, a PA can be obtained if other endocrine issues are present, such as cardiovascular risk, hypertension, heart disease, metabolic syndrome, unspecified cardiovascular risk, etc. Make sure your healthcare provider is aware of any diagnoses you may carry.

It's crucial to remember that off label use of medications should only be considered when the benefits outweigh the risks and under the supervision of your healthcare provider. These medications can have significant side effects and may not be suitable for everyone. Additionally, the effectiveness of these medications for weight loss can vary greatly among individuals. When choosing off label medications, it may be helpful in obtaining medications to omit the obesity code. Discuss this with your healthcare provider.

# Weight Gain Medications

## Medications that Cause Weight Gain

Many medications can potentially cause weight gain as a side effect. This weight gain can result from changes in appetite, metabolism, or fluid retention associated with these drugs. Here's a list of common types of medications that are known to possibly cause weight gain:

### Antidepressants

- **Selective Serotonin Reuptake Inhibitors (SSRIs)** such as Paroxetine (Paxil, Pexeva, Brisdelle), Sertraline (Zoloft), and Citalopram (Celexa).
- **Tricyclic Antidepressants (TCAs)** such as Amitriptyline, Doxepin, and Nortriptyline (Pamelor).
- **Atypical Antidepressants** like Mirtazapine (Remeron).

### Antipsychotics

- **Older Antipsychotics** (Typicals) such as Chlorpromazine and Haloperidol.
- **Newer Antipsychotics** (Atypicals) including Olanzapine (Zyprexa), Clozapine (Clozaril), and Quetiapine (Seroquel).

### Mood Stabilizers

- Drugs used for bipolar disorder like Lithium, Valproic Acid (Depakote), and Carbamazepine (Tegretol).

### Steroids

- Corticosteroids such as Prednisone and Methylprednisolone can cause significant weight gain when used for long periods.

### Anti-Seizure Drugs

- Medications like Gabapentin (Neurontin), Pregabalin (Lyrica), and Valproic Acid (Depakote).

# Weight Gain Medications

## Medications that Cause Weight Gain (continued)

### Diabetes Medications
- Insulin and insulin-related products often lead to weight gain.
- Sulfonylureas like Glyburide (Diabeta, Glynase) and Glipizide (Glucotrol).
- Thiazolidinediones such as Pioglitazone (Actos) and Rosiglitazone (Avandia).

### Beta Blockers
- Used for high blood pressure, such as Propranolol (Inderal), Metoprolol (Lopressor, Toprol XL), and Atenolol.

### Antihistamines
- Commonly used for allergies; medications like Diphenhydramine (Benadryl) and Cetirizine (Zyrtec) can increase appetite, thus leading to weight gain.

### Hormonal Medications
- Including birth control pills and hormone replacement therapy which can affect weight.

### Other Drugs
- Some antiretroviral drugs used to treat HIV
- Migraine and headache medications like Cyproheptadine
- Certain high blood pressure medications such as Prazosin and Clonidine

**What To Do**
If you think that your medication may be causing weight gain, discuss this with your healthcare provider. **Do not stop taking any medication without instructions from your healthcare provider.** Your doctor might adjust your dosage or prescribe to an alternative medication that does not have a significant impact on your weight.

## Authorization

To obtain prior authorization from an insurance company for off-label use of medication, you typically need to follow these steps:

- **Medical Necessity Documentation:** Your healthcare provider should give detailed documentation of your medical history and current condition, explaining why the off-label use of the medication is medically necessary. This may include clinical notes, treatment history, and any supporting evidence from medical literature or guidelines that justify the off-label use.

- **Specific Medication and Dosage:** Your healthcare provider should clearly specify the medication, its dosage, frequency, and duration of treatment. This must be precise to ensure the insurance company understands what is being requested.

- **Failure of Standard Treatments: Your provider should** document any standard treatments that have been tried and failed or if there are reasons they cannot be used (e.g., contraindications or side effects). This helps justify why an off-label option is being considered.

- **Prior Authorization Form:** Complete the insurance company's specific prior authorization form. This form usually requires information about you, the prescribing physician, and detailed medication information. It's important to answer all sections thoroughly. Any sections left blank will cause immediate denial.

- **Supporting Evidence:** Attach any supporting clinical evidence or peer-reviewed studies that support the efficacy and safety of the medication for specific off-label use. This could include case studies, articles from medical journals, or guidelines from reputable medical organizations.

## Authorization (continued)

- **Letter of Medical Justification:** Some insurers may require a letter from the physician that outlines the rationale for the off-label use, detailing how it is expected to benefit the patient's condition and why it is necessary over other treatments.

## Follow Up:

After submitting the request, keep track of its status and be prepared to provide additional information or clarification if the insurance company has questions or requires further documentation.

- **Appeal Process**
  In case the prior authorization is denied, be aware of the insurance company's appeal process. This usually involves submitting additional documentation or information to support the necessity of the treatment.

  - Review the denial letter thoroughly. It should specify the reason for denial (e.g., the medication isn't on their formulary, step therapy requirements, insufficient documentation, etc.).

  - If the reason is not clear, contact your insurance company.

  - Keep in mind that understanding the reason for denial is actually a blueprint for getting approval. Stay positive!

## Follow Up: (continued)

- **Provide Supporting Documentation**

  Work with your healthcare provider to submit additional documentation, Such as:

  - A letter of medical necessity explaining why a GLP-1 medication is essential for managing your disease and why alternatives are not suitable.

  - Keep in mind that understanding the reason for denial is actually a blueprint for getting approval. Stay positive!

  - Clinical records showing your history and current treatment regimen, A1C levels, BMI, and other relevant lab results.

  - Documentation of previous medication failures, adverse reactions, or lack of efficacy with other treatments.

  - For some insurance, only a diabetic diagnosis is the only allowable criteria. Some insurances cover prediabetes but very few.

It's beneficial to be thorough and provide as much detailed, supportive information as possible to increase the likelihood of approval. The process can vary slightly between insurance companies, so it's advisable to contact the specific insurer for their exact requirements and procedures.

It's crucial to remember that off-label use of medications should only be considered when the benefits outweigh the risks and under the supervision of your healthcare provider. These medications can have significant side effects and may not be suitable for everyone. Additionally, the effectiveness of these medications for weight loss can vary greatly among individuals. When choosing off-label medications, it may be helpful, in obtaining medications, to omit the obesity code. Discuss this with your healthcare provider.

# Step Therapy

## What is Step Therapy?

**Step therapy** is a cost-management strategy used by insurance companies to control the prescribing of medications, particularly newer and more expensive medications. In essence, step therapy requires you to first try one or more lower-cost or preferred medications often generic versions or older drugs before "stepping up" to a more expensive or newer medication, such as a GLP-1 agonist. If these initial treatments prove ineffective, intolerable, or unsuitable for you. Only then is the more costly medication covered by the insurance plan.

**The Rationale Behind Step Therapy** The primary goal of step therapy is to ensure that you receive the most cost-effective treatment that is appropriate for your condition. The rationale for implementing step therapy includes several key factors:

- **Cost Containment:**
  - **Managing Healthcare Costs:** Newer medications, especially those like GLP-1 agonists used in the management of type 2 diabetes and obesity, are often significantly more expensive than older treatments. By requiring you to try less expensive alternatives first, insurance companies aim to control overall healthcare spending.
  
  - **Encouraging the Use of Generics:** Generic medications, which are typically cheaper than brand-name drugs, are often preferred in step therapy protocols. This helps reduce the financial burden on both the healthcare system and you.

## What is Step Therapy?

**Step therapy** is a cost-management strategy used by insurance companies to control the prescribing of medications, particularly newer and more expensive medications. In essence, step therapy requires you to first try one or more lower-cost or preferred medications often generic versions or older drugs before "stepping up" to a more expensive or newer medication, such as a GLP-1 agonist. If these initial treatments prove ineffective, intolerable, or unsuitable for you. Only then is the more costly medication covered by the insurance plan.

**The Rationale Behind Step Therapy** The primary goal of step therapy is to ensure that you receive the most cost-effective treatment that is appropriate for your condition. The rationale for implementing step therapy includes several key factors:

- **Cost Containment:**
  - **Managing Healthcare Costs:** Newer medications, especially those like GLP-1 agonists used in the management of type 2 diabetes and obesity, are often significantly more expensive than older treatments. By requiring you to try less expensive alternatives first, insurance companies aim to control overall healthcare spending.

  - **Encouraging the Use of Generics:** Generic medications, which are typically cheaper than brand-name drugs, are often preferred in step therapy protocols. This helps reduce the financial burden on both the healthcare system and you.

# Step Therapy

## The Rationale Behind Step Therapy (continued)

While step therapy is designed to optimize healthcare spending and ensure effective treatment, it can also be a source of frustration for you and providers. You may experience delays in accessing the medications that ultimately may work best for you. Healthcare providers must navigate the often complex approval process. Despite these challenges, understanding the rationale behind step therapy can help you and your provider work more effectively within the system to achieve the best possible outcomes.

Before a person can obtain approval for a GLP-1 medication, insurance companies typically require that you try a series of other, often less expensive, treatments. These steps can vary depending on your specific condition (e.g., type 2 diabetes or obesity) and the insurance plan's policies. However, the most common treatments that must be tried before a GLP-1 medication include:

- **Lifestyle Interventions**
  - **Diet and Exercise:** You are usually required to attempt lifestyle changes, including a healthier diet and increased physical activity, as the first line of treatment, especially in cases of obesity or type 2 diabetes. These interventions are considered foundational for managing both conditions and can sometimes be enough to control symptoms without medication.

- **Metformin (For Type 2 Diabetes)**
  - **First-Line Medication:** Metformin is the most commonly prescribed initial medication for type 2 diabetes. It is inexpensive, widely available, and has a long history of effectiveness in lowering blood glucose levels. You are often required to use metformin and demonstrate that it is either insufficient in managing your blood sugar levels or that you experience intolerable side effects before being considered for GLP-1 medications.

## The Rationale Behind Step Therapy (continued)

- **Sulfonylureas**
  - **Alternative Oral Medications:** Sulfonylureas, such as glipizide or glyburide, are another class of oral medications used to manage blood sugar in type 2 diabetes. These medications stimulate the pancreas to produce more insulin. Insurers may require you to try these drugs if metformin alone is not effective before approving a GLP-1 receptor agonist.

- **DPP-4 Inhibitors**
  - **Incretin-Based Therapy:** DPP-4 inhibitors, such as sitagliptin (Januvia), are oral medications that help increase insulin production and decrease glucose production in the liver. They are often considered a step before GLP-1 receptor agonists because they work through a similar pathway but are generally less expensive and administered orally.

- **SGLT-2 Inhibitors**
  - **Newer Oral Agents:** Sodium-glucose co-transporter 2 (SGLT-2) inhibitors, like empagliflozin (Jardiance) and canagliflozin (Invokana), are another class of edications that may be required before moving to GLP-1 therapies. These drugs help lower blood glucose by causing the kidneys to excrete glucose in the urine.

- **Insulin Therapy**
  - **For Advanced Diabetes:** In some cases, particularly when diabetes is not well-controlled by oral medications, insulin therapy may be required before GLP-1 medications are considered. Insurers may want to ensure that a patient has attempted insulin, particularly long-acting or basal insulin, to see if it can effectively manage blood sugar levels.

# Step Therapy

## The Rationale Behind Step Therapy (continued)

- **Behavioral or Psychological Interventions**
  - **Especially in Obesity Management:** you may be required to try other weight loss medications, such as orlistat, phentermine, or naltrexone/bupropion (Contrave), before moving on to a GLP-1 medication like semaglutide or Tirzepatide, especially if the primary indication is obesity.

- **Previous Use of Weight Loss Medications**
  - **For Obesity:** If you are seeking GLP-1 medications for weight management, insurers might require that you participate in behavioral counseling or other psychological interventions aimed at changing your eating habits or addressing underlying psychological factors contributing to obesity. GLP-1 medications that are not FDA-approved for weight loss, in most cases will be denied. Other diagnoses must be considered such as metabolic syndrome, increased risk of cardiac events, insulin resistance, etc.

- **Your History and Documentation**
  - **Proof of Inefficacy or Intolerance:** Your healthcare provider will need to provide documentation showing that the aforementioned treatments were either ineffective or caused intolerable side effects. This documentation often includes medical records, prescription history, and notes from healthcare providers.

These steps ensure that GLP-1 medications are prescribed appropriately and only after other, potentially less costly, treatments have been tried and found insufficient. It's important for you and your provider to understand these requirements to navigate the approval process successfully.

## Obtaining Medications From A Compound Pharmacy

Compound pharmacies are a great resource for customizing medications to fit your specific needs. If a medication appears on the FDA drug shortage list, regulations are relaxed, and compounding pharmacies can produce medications that cannot be obtained.

- **Function:** Unlike regular pharmacies that dispense mass-produced medications, compound pharmacies create custom formulations.
  This can involve:
  - **Altering dosage:** Maybe a standard dosage is too strong or needs splitting for a child.
  - **Changing form:** A medication that comes in pill form might be better tolerated as a cream if swallowing is difficult.
  - **Combining medications:** This can simplify your regimen by putting multiple meds into one.
  - **Addressing allergies:** If you have allergies to inactive ingredients in a commercial medication, a compound pharmacy can create one without the allergens.

- **Governance:** There are two main types of compound pharmacies with different regulations:
  - **503A Compounding Pharmacies:** These are state-licensed and primarily fulfill prescriptions from individual doctors for specific patients.
  - **503B Compounding Pharmacies:** These are FDA-approved facilities that can mass-produce compounded medications and distribute them to hospitals or other healthcare providers. mass-produce compounded medications and distribute them to hospitals or other healthcare providers.

# Compound Pharmacy

## Obtaining Medications From A Compound Pharmacy (continued)

- **Safety:** The safety of compounded medications can vary depending on the pharmacy. Here's what to consider:

  - **Use a reputable pharmacy:** Look for pharmacies with a history of quality control and adherence to USP (United States Pharmacopeia) standards.

  - **Work with the pharmacist:** Your healthcare provider should discuss your specific needs with the pharmacy. Here's what to consider to ensure the compounded medication is appropriate.

  - **Be aware of limitations:** Compounded medications haven't undergone the same rigorous testing as commercially available drugs. Their effectiveness and potential side effects may not be fully established.

**Overall, compound pharmacies can be a valuable tool for providing customized medications. However, it's important to understand the regulatory landscape and work with a reputable pharmacy to ensure your safety.**

Here are some resources for you to learn more:

- **International Academy of Compounding Pharmacists (IACP):** https://uia.org/s/or/en/1100023143

- **FDA's Guidance for 503A Compounding:** https://www.fda.gov/files/drugs/published/Compounded-Drug-Products-That-Are-Essentially-Copies-of-a-Commercially-Available-Drug-Product-Under-Section-503A-of-the-Federal-Food--Drug--and-Cosmetic-Act-Guidance-for-Industry.pdf

# Health Benefits Of Losing Weight By Percentage

When you lose weight, even modest amounts can lead to significant health improvements. Here's how losing different percentages of your body weight can impact your health:

## Losing 5% of Your Body Weight

**Cardiovascular Health:** Blood pressure tends to decrease, reducing the risk of heart disease. LDL cholesterol (bad cholesterol) and triglyceride levels often drop, while HDL cholesterol (good cholesterol) may increase.

**Blood Sugar Levels:** Insulin sensitivity improves, which can lower the risk of developing type 2 diabetes. For those with type 2 diabetes, it may improve blood sugar control.

**Inflammation:** There's often a reduction in inflammatory markers, which can decrease the risk of chronic diseases.

**Joint Health:** Even a small amount of weight loss can reduce the stress on joints, especially in the knees, which can alleviate pain from conditions like osteoarthritis.

## Losing 10% of Your Body Weight

**Blood Pressure:** Further reduction in blood pressure, which may reduce the need for medications in some individuals.

**Blood Sugar and Insulin:** More pronounced improvements in blood sugar levels and insulin sensitivity, potentially leading to reduced reliance on diabetes medications.

**Liver Health:** Continued improvements in cholesterol levels, with further reductions in LDL and triglycerides and an increase in HDL.

**Joint Health:** Reduced risk of non-alcoholic fatty liver disease (NAFLD) and potential reversal of early-stage liver damage.

**Mobility and Joint Pain:** Noticeable improvement in mobility and a further reduction in joint pain, enhancing overall quality of life.

# Health Benefits

## Health Benefits Of Losing Weight By Percentage
(continued)

### Losing 15% of Your Body Weight

**Metabolic Health:** Substantial improvements in metabolic health, including lower risk of metabolic syndrome, which includes conditions like high blood pressure, high blood sugar, excess body fat around the waist, and abnormal cholesterol levels.

**Cardiovascular Risk:** Significant reduction in cardiovascular risk, potentially lowering the risk of heart attacks and strokes.

**Inflammation:** Greater reduction in systemic inflammation, which is linked to a variety of chronic conditions.

**Respiratory Function:** Improved lung function can be especially beneficial for individuals with sleep apnea or asthma.

**Energy Levels:** Noticeable energy and physical stamina increase, making engaging in physical activities easier.

### Losing 20% of Your Body Weight

**Overall Mortality Risk:** A significant reduction in the risk of premature death from obesity-related conditions such as heart disease, stroke, and certain cancers.

**Hormonal Balance:** Improved hormonal balance, particularly in individuals with polycystic ovary syndrome (PCOS).

**Kidney Function:** Reduced risk of chronic kidney disease, particularly in those with diabetes or hypertension.

**Mental Health:** Potential improvements in mood, self-esteem, and overall mental well-being, and a reduced risk of depression.

**Mobility:** Drastic improvement in mobility and quality of life, significantly reduced joint pain and increased ease of movement.

## Health Benefits Of Losing Weight By Percentage
*(continued)*

### Losing 30% of Your Body Weight

**Cardiovascular Health:** significantly reducing the risk of cardiovascular events such as heart attacks and strokes. Blood pressure, cholesterol, and triglyceride levels may normalize, reducing the need for medication.

**Diabetes Management:** For individuals with type 2 diabetes, a 30% weight loss can lead to substantial improvements, including the potential for remission of the disease. Insulin sensitivity can be greatly enhanced, and the need for diabetes medications may be significantly reduced or eliminated.

**Liver and Kidney Health:** Further reductions in liver fat, potentially reversing non-alcoholic fatty liver disease (NAFLD) and improving liver function. Kidney function can also improve, reducing the risk of chronic kidney disease.

**Joint and Bone Health:** Dramatic reduction in stress on joints, which can alleviate or even eliminate pain from osteoarthritis and improve overall mobility. Bone density may improve as the body's inflammatory markers decrease.

**Respiratory and Sleep Health:** Major improvements in conditions like sleep apnea and asthma lead to better sleep quality and increased energy during the day.

**Hormonal and Reproductive Health:** Significant improvements in hormonal balance, especially in conditions like polycystic ovary syndrome (PCOS). Fertility may improve, and menstrual cycles may become more regular.

# Health Benefits

## Health Benefits Of Losing Weight By Percentage
(continued)

### Losing 30% of Your Body Weight
(continued)

**Mental and Emotional Health:** Marked improvements in mental health, including reduced symptoms of depression and anxiety. Self-esteem and body image can improve significantly, leading to a better overall quality of life.

**Cancer Risk:** A substantial reduction in the risk of obesity-related cancers, such as breast, colon, and endometrial cancers.

**Longevity:** A 30% weight loss can extend life expectancy by reducing the risk of obesity-related diseases and improving overall health.

## Conclusion:

Each step of weight loss, whether **5%, 10%, 15%**, or **20%**, brings its own set of health benefits, progressively reducing the risk of chronic diseases, improving metabolic function, and enhancing overall well-being. At **30%,** weight loss represents a transformative change, providing profound health benefits across almost all systems of the body. It significantly lowers the risk of chronic diseases, enhances physical and mental well-being, and can lead to a much-improved quality of life and increased longevity.

# Health Benefits
## of GLP-1 and GLP-1/GIL Medications

Both Semaglutide and Tirzepatide contribute to improvements in metabolic health and the management of chronic diseases in several ways:

### Metabolic Syndrome

**Semaglutide**

**Insulin resistance:** By enhancing insulin secretion in response to meals and reducing glucagon secretion, Semaglutide improves insulin sensitivity, which is a central issue in Metabolic Syndrome.

**Obesity:** Significant weight loss facilitated by semaglutide can directly reduce obesity, a major criterion of Metabolic Syndrome.

**Lipid Profiles:** Treatment with Semaglutide has been shown to improve lipid profiles, reduce levels of LDL cholesterol and triglycerides, and sometimes increase HDL cholesterol.

**Blood Pressure:** While not a primary effect, reductions in blood pressure have been observed in some individuals, likely secondary to weight loss and improved insulin sensitivity.

## Health Benefits
## of GLP-1 and GLP-1/GIL Medications (continued)

### Metabolic Syndrome (continued)

**Tirzepatide**

**Insulin Resistance:** The combination of GLP-1 and GIP action helps improve insulin sensitivity and glycemic control more effectively than GLP-1 alone.

**Weight Reduction:** Tirzepatide has been shown to result in notable weight loss, addressing the central obesity component of Metabolic Syndrome

**Lipld Profiles**: Individuals using Tirzepatide have reported improvements in their lipid profiles, which contribute to reducing the cardiovascular risk associated with Metabolic Syndrome.

**Blood Pressure Effects:** As with Semaglutide, Tirzepatide may also lead to improvements in blood pressure, especially beneficial for those with high blood pressure as part of their Metabolic Syndrome diagnosis.

Both of these medications contribute to a holistic approach to managing Metabolic Syndrome, not only by targeting blood sugar levels but also by improving Metabolic health markers and overall cardiovascular risk. This makes them valuable in treating individuals with complex metabolic health profiles.

# Health Benefits
## of GLP-1 and GLP-1/GIL Medications (continued)

### Gut Microbiota

**Semaglutide**: There is emerging evidence that GLP-1 agonists like Semaglutide can affect the composition and function of the gut microbiota. These changes are believed to be beneficial, potentially promoting a more favorable gut flora profile that can enhance metabolic health and immune function. The mechanism may involve alterations in gut motility and nutrient absorption, which can indirectly affect the growth and activity of different microbial populations.

**Tirzepatide:** Given its recent introduction and similar mechanism of action, Tirzepatide might also impact the gut microbiota. Its dual incretin effect could amplify these benefits, possibly promoting a diverse and stable microbial community that supports overall health. However, direct studies on Tirzepatide's effects on the gut microbiota are still required to confirm these effects.

### Alzheimer's Disease

**Semaglutide**: There is a growing interest in the role of insulin resistance in the brain and its association with Alzheimer's disease. As a GLP-1 receptor agonist, Semaglutide could potentially benefit cognitive functions by improving brain insulin signaling and reducing neuroinflammation. Preliminary studies in animal models suggest that GLP-1 agonists might reduce amyloid and tau phosphorylation, which are hallmarks of Alzheimer's pathology.

**Tirzepatide:** While specific research on Tirzepatide and Alzheimer's disease is limited, its effect on brain health could be hypothesized, given the known benefits of GLP-1 receptor activation in neuroprotective pathways. The combination of GLP-1 and GIP effects might offer additional advantages in modulating brain metabolism and inflammation.

## Health Benefits
## of GLP-1 and GLP-1/GIL Medications (continued)

### Chronic Kidney Disease (CKD)

**Semaglutide:** It can improve various components of metabolic syndrome, including blood pressure, lipid profiles, and waist circumference, alongside its effects on blood glucose and body weight.

**Tirzepatide:** Similarly, by improving glycemic control and aiding in substantial weight loss, Tirzepatide can reduce blood pressure and lipid levels, contributing to a reduction in the overall risk of metabolic syndrome.

### Sleep Apnea

**Semaglutide:** By significantly reducing weight, Semaglutide may improve symptoms of sleep apnea in patients with obesity, as weight loss is often recommended to alleviate sleep apnea symptoms.

**Tirzepatide:** Given its efficacy in weight reduction, Tirzepatide may also help in reducing the severity of sleep apnea, though direct studies are needed to confirm these effects.

## Health Benefits of GLP-1 and GLP-1/GIL Medications (continued)

### Chronic Inflammation

**Semaglutide:** There is emerging evidence that GLP-1 agonists like Semaglutide may have anti-inflammatory properties, which could be beneficial in various chronic diseases characterized by inflammation.

**Tirzepatide:** Its dual mechanism action may also confer anti-inflammatory effects, potentially impacting conditions like cardiovascular diseases and metabolic disorders that have an inflammatory component.

Both medications have profound effects on systemic health. They not only influence primary disease processes for which they are prescribed but also provide ancillary benefits that can improve overall chronic disease management and quality of life.

## Health Benefits
## of GLP-1 and GLP-1/GIL Medications (continued)

**The benefits of Semaglutide and Tirzepatide extend into areas like mental health (depression), reproductive health (PCOS), and chronic inflammatory conditions (Rheumatoid Arthritis), though research in these fields is still developing:**

### Depression

**Semaglutide:** Emerging research suggests that GLP-1 agonists might have a beneficial impact on mental health, including depression. This is possibly due to the improvement in metabolic health and weight management, which can significantly affect mental well-being. There's also a hypothesis about direct effects on brain function and mood regulation through GLP-1 receptors in the brain.

**Tirzepatide:** While specific studies on Tirzepatide and depression are limited, the potential for mental health benefits similar to those of Semaglutide exists, given the overall improvements in physical health and metabolic states that can influence mood and quality of life.

### Polycystic Ovary Syndrome (PCOS)

**Semaglutide:** The weight loss associated with Semaglutide can help manage PCOS symptoms, primarily by improving insulin resistance, a key issue in PCOS. Weight loss can also help restore ovulatory cycles and improve fertility in women with PCOS.

**Tirzepatide:** Given its potent effects on weight reduction and potential improvements in insulin sensitivity, Tirzepatide could be beneficial in managing PCOS, though direct research is still needed.

## Health Benefits
## of GLP-1 and GLP-1/GIL Medications (continued)

The benefits of Semaglutide and Tirzepatide extend into areas like mental health (depression), reproductive health (PCOS), and chronic inflammatory conditions (Rheumatoid Arthritis), though research in these fields is still developing:

### Rheumatoid Arthritis (RA)

**Semaglutide:** There is interest in the potential anti-inflammatory properties of GLP-1 agonists like Semaglutide that could indirectly benefit inflammatory diseases like RA. However, direct evidence linking semaglutide to improvements in RA symptoms is currently lacking.

**Tirzepatide:** Similarly, while the anti-inflammatory effects of Tirzepatide could theoretically benefit RA, research directly examining this connection is not yet available.

## Health Benefits
## of GLP-1 and GLP-1/GIL Medications (continued)

### Pain Management

**Semaglutide:** There is limited but intriguing evidence suggesting that GLP-1 receptor agonists may have an analgesic effect, potentially due to their anti-inflammatory properties and effects on neural pathways. For example, some studies have reported reduced neuropathic pain in diabetic peripheral neuropathy, which could be mediated by improved glycemic control and reduced systemic inflammation.

**Tirzepatide:** As a newer drug, direct studies on Tirzepatide's impact on pain are scarce. However, given its potent effects on inflammation and metabolic improvement, it might also contribute to pain reduction, particularly in conditions associated with obesity and metabolic syndrome.

### Psoriasis

**Semaglutide:** While there are no direct studies linking Semaglutide to improvements in psoriasis, the drug's potential anti-inflammatory effects could theoretically benefit inflammatory skin conditions like psoriasis. Psoriasis is often associated with metabolic syndrome, and improving metabolic health could indirectly benefit skin health.

**Tirzepatide:** Similarly, the potential for Tirzepatide to impact psoriasis would likely stem from its effects on systemic inflammation and metabolic health. Improved insulin sensitivity and reduced adiposity might decrease the systemic inflammation that exacerbates psoriasis.

For both pain and psoriasis, the evidence remains speculative and largely inferential based on the known mechanisms of action of these medications and their effects on related conditions. Future research may uncover more definitive links and potentially expand the therapeutic uses of semaglutide and Tirrzepatide to include these areas.

## Talking Points for Your HealthCare Provider

When discussing weight loss medications with your doctor, it's important to have an open and honest conversation. Here are some key talking points that you may want to consider:

- **Weight Loss History:**
  - Provide a detailed history of your past attempts at weight loss, including any diets, exercise programs, or lifestyle changes you've tried.
  - Mention any challenges or obstacles you've faced in achieving and maintaining a healthy weight.

- **Current Health Status:**
  - Discuss your current health status, including any existing medical conditions, medications you are currently taking, and any recent changes in your health.
  - Inform your doctor about any concerns or symptoms related to your weight, such as joint pain, fatigue, or difficulty with physical activities.

- **Nutritional Habits:**
  - Describe your typical eating habits, including the types of foods you consume, portion sizes, and frequency of meals.
  - Mention any emotional or stress-related eating patterns you may have and how they affect your weight.

- **Physical Activity:**
  - Talk about your current level of physical activity, including the type, duration, and frequency of exercise you engage in.
  - Discuss any barriers or challenges you face in maintaining an active lifestyle.

# Talking Points for Your HealthCare Provider
(continued)

- **Psychosocial Factors:**
  - Share information about any emotional or psychological factors that may contribute to your weight gain or make weight loss challenging.
  - Discuss stress levels, emotional well-being, and any factors that may influence your ability to make healthy lifestyle choices.

- **Weight Loss Goals:**
  - Clearly communicate your weight loss goals to your doctor, including both short-term and long-term goals.
  - Be realistic about what you hope to achieve and the timeline you have in mind.

- **Knowledge about Medications:**
  - Express any knowledge or concerns you have about weight loss medications.
  - Ask your doctor to provide information about the potential benefits, risks, and side effects of the medications under consideration.

- **Questions and Concerns:**
  - Prepare a list of questions and concerns you may have about weight loss medications.
  - Inquire about alternative approaches, if any, that your doctor recommends or thinks may be suitable for you.

Remember, the discussion with your doctor should be a collaborative effort, and it's important to work together to find the most appropriate and effective solution for your individual needs and health conditions.

# Summary

**In this comprehensive guide,** we have explored the multifaceted landscape of weight loss medications, providing insights into how their function, their benefits, potential side effects, and the vital role they can play in the journey towards a healthier life. The decision to embark on a weight loss journey using medication is significant and should not be taken lightly. It requires careful consideration, a deep understanding of the options available, and, most importantly, a commitment to ongoing health and wellness.

As we conclude, remember that weight loss medications are tools, not cures. They are most effective when used along with a balanced diet, regular physical activity, and positive lifestyle changes. I encourage you to take what you've learned here and engage in an open, informed dialogue with your healthcare provider to determine the best path forward tailored to your personal health needs and goals.

**Take action today!** Reach out to your healthcare professional, discuss your options, and take the first step towards a healthier, more vibrant you. The journey may be challenging, but the rewards of improved health and well-being are worth every step.

**Remember, every journey begins with one step. Take yours today!**

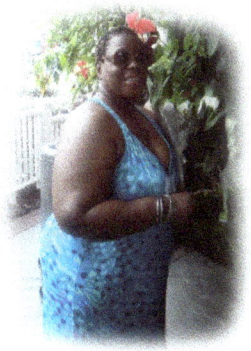 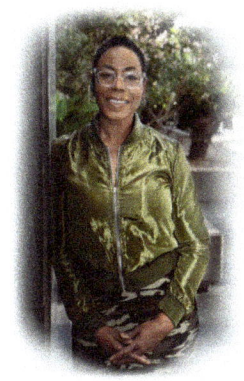

## Bibliography

- *Drucker, D. J. (2006). The biology of incretin hormones. Cell Metabolism, 3(3), 153-165.*

- *Mannucci, E., et al. (2010). GLP-1 receptor agonists for the treatment of type 2 diabetes: A review of the evidence. Diabetes, Obesity and Metabolism, 12(8), 641-647.*

- *Garvey, W. T., et al. (2016). American Association of Clinical Endocrinologists and American College of Endocrinology comprehensive clinical practice guidelines for medical care of patients with obesity. Endocrine Practice, 22(Suppl 3), 1-203.*

- *U.S. Food and Drug Administration. (2021). FDA Approves Wegovy (semaglutide) for Chronic Weight Management in Adults.*

- *Anderson, S. L., & Trujillo, J. M. (2015). Liraglutide for chronic weight management: A review of the literature and safety considerations. Pharmacy and Therapeutics, 40(11), 812-818.*

- *Nauck, M. A., et al. (2017). Risks and benefits of GLP-1 receptor agonists: A focus on cardiovascular outcomes. Diabetes, Obesity and Metabolism, 19(3), 285-294.*

- *Sullivan, S. D., et al. (2019). The role of health insurance in obesity treatment. Obesity Research & Clinical Practice, 13(6), 531-538.*

- *U.S. Government Accountability Office. (2019). Obesity drugs: Few adults used prescription drugs for weight loss, and insurance coverage varied. GAO-19-207.*

- *Astrup, A., & Finer, N. (2000). Redefining Type 2 diabetes: 'Diabesity' or obesity dependent diabetes mellitus? Obesity Reviews, 1(1), 57-59.*

- *Pi-Sunyer, F. X. (1993). Medical hazards of obesity. Annals of Internal Medicine, 119 (7 Pt 2), 655-660.*

## Bibliography (continued)

- *Kelly, A. S., et al. (2022). A randomized, controlled trial of semaglutide in adolescents with obesity. New England Journal of Medicine, 387, 224-232.*

- *Wing, R. R., & Phelan, S. (2005). Long-term weight loss maintenance. American Journal of Clinical Nutrition, 82(1), 222S-225S.*

- *Wadden, T. A., et al. (2011). Behavioral treatment of obesity in patients encountered in primary care settings: A systematic review. JAMA, 312(17), 1779-1791.*

www.ingramcontent.com/pod-product-compliance
Lightning Source LLC
Chambersburg PA
CBHW070541030426
42337CB00016B/2306